# A Fat Girl's Manifesto

# Advanced Praise for Cyr Daniel's *A Fat Girl's Manifesto*

Cyr V. Daniel's *A Fat Girl's Manifesto* is educational and uplifting. Daniel introduces her audience to current research on weight and health with wit and simplicity. The old paradigm—fat is bad, and you must lose weight to be healthy—is not supported by scientific evidence. Daniel is an admirer of the work of Glenn Gaesser (including his groundbreaking book, Big Fat Lies), using quotes from that book to illustrate her points.

In between the quotes, Daniel's unique voice comes through. She describes her journey towards self-acceptance in an honest and entertaining way. She critiques the traditional view of weight with clever humor. Given the adage "Being fat will shorten your life," Daniel says that would be true if you add two words to the phrase—namely, "in America." In her words, "Living in a country where you are bombarded with officially sanctioned anti-fat sentiments everywhere you turn is extremely stressful, and people... stress kills!"

Her personal testimony includes the pain of lectures on weight from her father; the shame of overhearing her parents argue about who was to blame for their daughter's weight; and her feeling as a young girl that life was unfair. It will be all too familiar to many people who grew up in any of the past few decades. But then Cyr's journey takes a turn. She is an artist, with a degree in sculpture and ceramics. And while in college, she decided to be brave and become an artist's model. Posing nude for art students—and becoming a much-requested model—gave her an appreciation of her body that no amount of reading and research can provide.

Cyr Daniel tells her readers how she reclaimed her body and her life. She still encounters prejudice, but she has the self-esteem to fend it off. When a thin woman treats her with contempt, Cyr now understands that the contempt often comes from that woman's own struggle with self-love. She writes:

*A friend of mine posted these words where she would see them every day:*

*"Nothing tastes as good as thin feels"*

Words to live by? For me...not so much. If most men lead lives of quiet desperation, most women (in this culture at least) lead lives of quiet deprivation.

I do have one quibble with the book. Daniel feels that the airlines have the right to charge larger people for two seats. As an activist against weight discrimination, I have worked on this problem for many years. It might be legitimate to base freight costs on the size and weight of a piece of cargo, but airlines carry people, not freight. They charge to transport one person from point A to point B. They do not charge less for children or very thin people. So I have to disagree with Cyr Daniel on this issue.

*A Fat Girl's Manifesto* provides a good balance between science and personal testimony. Daniel offers an easy-to understand summary of the latest research: being heavier than average is not as bad as you think, and restrictive dieting and weight obsession are neither effective nor healthful. Her spirited personality shines through as she relates her journey towards self-acceptance. The book is a pleasant and worthwhile read.

***—Miriam Berg, President of The Council on Size and Weight Discrimination***

*A Fat Girl's Manifesto* should be required reading for every health, wellness and fitness professional, regardless of if they work with the overweight population or not. With sharp insight, humor and candidness, Cyr opens the window for the reader to glimpse through and see what it is like growing up and living in America in a body which society deems as too big and unhealthy.

Based on a foundation of solid research and science, this book will strip away any ill-founded assumptions and preconceived notions you might have, and clearly shows that you can, contrary to popular belief, be fat and fit. It is time for everyone, including the diet and fitness industry, to stop profiting from the vulnerability and insecurities of the overweight. Let's produce products and services that emphasize health, not weight loss, as a primary goal, and do so with compassion, respect and dignity.

***—Ellen G. Goldman, M.Ed., Certified Professional Wellness Coach, Certified Personal Trainer, EnerGcoaching.com***

This is a little book with a big message. Regardless of our size, accepting ourselves is fundamental to truly understanding what each of us needs for health and happiness. Kudos to Cyr Daniel for discovering that for herself and spreading the message.

***—Marsha Hudnall, MS, RDN, CD, President & Co-Owner, Green Mountain at Fox Run***

Cyr Daniel says, "I can't tell you how many women I've seen—fat and thin—obsessed with dieting and hating their perfectly beautiful bodies. It strikes me as a sad way to spend life's precious moments."

A woman whose life was similarly oppressed by antifat prejudice, Daniel broke free. She learned what she calls the TRUTH* behind the FIBs and FIB2s that underlie the oppression. With an engaging sense of humor and a knack for useful acronyms, she encourages 'consciousness fattening' in the reader. She makes several good points, such as the economic costs of fat prejudice vs. those of sports, exercise, and recreation.

This quick, easy read demonstrates her long-held decision that her life would never be about quantity, but always about quality. It's easy to see from her photo and her story that she chooses "friends, fun, and food every time." *Read the book to decode the acronyms.

***—Barbara Altman Bruno, PhD, LCSW, author,* Worth Your Weight**

You have been led to believe lies... in her often times witty and always brilliant memoir, Cyr Daniel shows us how to stop the self-loathing and see ourselves and our bodies in a new, much more sensible and intelligent way. This book gives new meaning to the old adage... change the way you see, not the way you look. Her book is a call for a revolution and awakening in the way people perceive themselves.

***—Lisa Sanders, Life Coach & Intuitive Consultant***

No overweight American should be scared to walk into a gym, regardless of social norm or media pressure. Cyr is an inspiration. A true revolutionary for one of the most misunderstood niches of the fitness industry. An amazing memoir by a brilliant fat-fit soul. Cyr provokes and challenges what was cut and dry fundamental in fitness and turns it upside down!

***—Michael Cupples, Certified Personal Trainer***

# A Fat Girl's Manifesto

## A thin book on living FAT in America

By

**Cyr V. Daniel**

2015
Peter E. Randall Publisher
Portsmouth, New Hampshire

ISBN: 978-1-931807-95-1
Library of Congress Control No.: 2014945376

Published by
Peter E. Randall Publisher
PO Box 4726
Portsmouth, NH 03802
www.perpublisher.com

Book design: Grace Peirce (nhmuse.com)



*Please note: This article was published more than one year ago. The facts and conclusions presented may have since changed and may no longer be accurate. And "More information" links may no longer work. Questions about personal health should always be referred to a physician or other health care professional.

# *Dedication*

This book is dedicated to my daughters first and foremost. You have always been and will always be my sun, moon, stars, and joy. It is also dedicated to all the people I love. You know who you are, and I am forever grateful for the happiness, wisdom, and love you share with me with such unparalleled generosity.

# *Acknowledgments*

I have to give a special all-star MVP acknowledgment to my dear friend Lisa Sanders. She has been after me to write a book for many years and became absolutely relentless in her urging once I retired. She was my first reader, is my most vocal and tireless supporter, and has lavished this project with her boundless energy and wisdom well beyond her years. I want to thank my other early readers for their eagle eyes, valued opinions and enthusiasm for the manuscript. My heartfelt appreciation to Jen Brown, Kim Cahill, Jeanne Currier, Lorraine DeYoung, Vallerie Dow, Audrey Giumarra, Jai Holly, Oleyemi Mahoney, Ellen Mason, Marge McGann, Brandy Mitroff, Deb Muir, Barry and Dottie Perlow, and Lori Worthen. Another thank you to Grace Peirce for juggling lots of ideas and one hefty ego (guess whose?) yet managing to create the wonderful cover design for this book. And finally, my thanks to Deidre Randall, my publisher, for her marvelous advice and judicious words of encouragement.

# *Contents*


Dedication . . . . . . . . . . . . . . . . . . . . . . . . . . . . ix
Acknowledgments . . . . . . . . . . . . . . . . . . . . . . . . xi
Introduction . . . . . . . . . . . . . . . . . . . . . . . . . . . xv
The Early Years . . . . . . . . . . . . . . . . . . . . . . . . . 1
The Current to Be Swum Against . . . . . . . . . . . . . . . 7
The TRUTH . . . . . . . . . . . . . . . . . . . . . . . . . . . 15
FIB$^2$s . . . . . . . . . . . . . . . . . . . . . . . . . . . . . 25
The Planet Fat . . . . . . . . . . . . . . . . . . . . . . . . . 41
The Choice—To BElieve or Not To BElieve . . . . . . . 49
The Home Stretch . . . . . . . . . . . . . . . . . . . . . . . 63
The Manifesto . . . . . . . . . . . . . . . . . . . . . . . . . 71
Bibliography . . . . . . . . . . . . . . . . . . . . . . . . . . 75
About the Author . . . . . . . . . . . . . . . . . . . . . . . 79
The "Skinny" on the About the Author Photo . . . . 80

# *Introduction*

Write about what you know. That's the first rule you will hear in about every writing class the world over. Well, there is one thing I know about better than any other: being fat in America from the 1950s to the present day.

I have had a blast writing this book. It's been waiting to come out for at least three decades, and getting it out of my head on to paper has been an exciting and enlightening experience. When you read some of the research I discovered along the way, you will understand why. But it is important for you to understand one thing with crystal clarity. I am not writing this book to make excuses or play a pity card. I am writing this to share with you the conclusions I have drawn after living sixty plus years fat in this society. It's about how I stopped believing that Fat Is Bad and found self-acceptance. For the rest of this book Fat is Bad will be represented by

FIB, since it is a whopping one and I don't even like typing out those words.

The FIB messages (see Chapter 4) came unwelcomed and often during my childhood, and they are still coming plentifully on a daily basis. From TV to newspaper articles to the Internet, this ubiquitous message is being drummed into my mind and yours as an irrefutable fact. It's the Eleventh Commandment of our culture. Thou Shalt Not Be Fat! Break that commandment and there will be consequences, but it doesn't make that statement a fact. I am here to tell you it is only an opinion, a pretty shaky one, too, when you start to look at the real facts, and one to which I no longer subscribe. This is the story of my journey from believing just about every negative theory on being fat to living fiercely, fearlessly, and most important, fabulously fat.

A cautionary note before you read further. I have oft been told by friends and family that I am a grandmaster at making a short story long. If this skill were an Olympic event, I would be team USA's best hope to bring home the gold.

Maybe it's because I believe "Bigger Is Better" in all good things. Translation: There will likely appear to be numerous digressions as I tell my story. Patiently meander along with me and I promise I'll tie most, if not all, of the loose ends together by the end.

OK. Enough with the introduction already. Let's get started!

CHAPTER 1

# *The Early Years*

I don't remember when I first became aware that I was fat and that to be so was a very bad thing indeed. It feels like I have always been aware of that opinion. I went from a plump baby to a child with "baby fat." My weight was never "normal" by the standards of the day, and the pounds just kept coming. In elementary school I was teased relentlessly and cruelly on a daily basis.

By high school I was pushing 200 pounds and had developed a cruel defense mechanism of my own. When attacked for my weight, I learned to strike back with a quick and vicious wit using burning sarcasm to point out my attacker's flaws. My reputation for rejoinders so cutting they drew psychological blood and so clever they became hall chatter for weeks soon made the teasing stop. The damage had been done though. I put up a great front, but my self-image was shattered. I cried a lot in the privacy of my bedroom and begged God to take the fat away.

I can still remember gathering around the television with my mom and dad to watch the "Miss America Pageant." In the 1950s and most of the 1960s (before the women's movement), the pageant was taken very seriously. The contestants represented the ideal American woman. The message wasn't lost on me. My tearful nightly bargains with God—and any power in the universe that might be willing to deliver me from the fat curse—were particularly heartfelt on pageant night.

My parents tried everything to get me to lose weight. I interpreted their constant efforts as proof they didn't really believe "It's what's inside that counts." I mean, they were preaching that saying out of the same mouths that were constantly telling me I had to lose weight if I wanted to be happy and succeed in life. Their mixed message may have been my first experience with "political correctness" even though that term wouldn't be coined for a few more decades.

To me the 50s and 60s weren't The Age of Aquarius. They were The Age of Hypocrisy. They were the *Ozzie & Harriet, Father Knows Best, Leave It to Beaver, Dick Van Dyke, Danny Thomas, Donna Reed Show* years. My family did a lot of playacting for the world, but when it was just us, it was made crystal clear that being fat was not a good thing.

They told me to cultivate my brain and my "great sense of humor" because I would "never be beautiful." I was told not to expect to have boyfriends or a husband and children. (Spoiler alert! I did have a husband and he was a handsome, brilliant renaissance man. Want proof I'm not just jiving? He taught Missile Guidance at West Point during his stint in the army and made my solid gold, coral motif (I collect coral) wedding ring from scratch. That is just a miniscule example of his range and depth of talents and knowledge. Handsome of course is in the eye of the beholder, but even my parents, who weren't one hundred percent in love with my husband because he didn't make enough money to suit them, thought he was handsome. I was also blessed with two amazing-in-every-way daughters.) I was told not to expect good medical care because doctors were reluctant to treat fat patients. I would have to give my parents some validity points on this one. I have dealt with docs who clearly have psychotic issues about dealing with fat people, but I quickly ran the other way. I have found plenty of great docs out there who have always shown me personal respect and given me excellent treatment. And I'm Jewish so I am an expert on judging doctors! I honestly can't remember all the crap they told me. I just remember the warnings about the myriad awful repercussions of being fat were endless.

Now, don't get me wrong here. My parents weren't monsters and I am not looking for sympathy or trying to jump on the "I had a traumatic childhood" bandwagon. They held our society's beliefs about the evils of being fat, and they tried everything from scare tactics to bribery to get me to diet. (Best bribe...I wanted a horse and they told me I could have one if I lost the weight.)

I was put on every diet that came down the pike. Among the endless diets were the grapefruit diet, the Metracal diet, and my personal favorite, the weekly visits to a quack diet doctor who gave me mystery injections to help me lose weight accompanied by mean-spirited lectures on all the health perils I was courting by my failure to do so.

I have come to believe that my parents' primary motivation was love, but I know for a fact that some of their motivation was shame. I can still remember the look on my mother's face when her friends with thin kids would give her a catty smile and condescendingly simper, "Don't worry Audrey, it's just baby fat" even when I was well into my teens. My mother was a great beauty, and it must have killed her on many levels to have a fat daughter. I am sure her society lady friends were jealous of her for many reasons, not just her astonishing good looks, and loved reminding her of her fat child.

To make matters exponentially worse, my father was the president of a chain of fine clothing stores. Think Macy's or Jordan Marsh and you will get the picture. The business had been started by his father, so the personal pride in the stores ran deep for him.

He dressed impeccably at all times (ate dinner in his suit and tie) to represent the store and expected my mother and me to do the same. This meant being well dressed in the latest fashions every day all day. Sounds like a dream come true to a lot of you ladies out there, I bet, but for me it was a nightmare.

I dreaded every shopping trip to my father's store because none of the children's clothes fit me. (I was in my teens before a fashion line came out for fatties. It was called Chubette Fashions but was too little too late for me.) I spent hours in the fitting room surrounded by mirrors and standing on a raised platform while two gray-haired women who worked in the alterations department scuttled around on their knees, mouths full of pins, hemming up dresses that were way too long because they were adult sizes.

There were endless discussions of how many inches seams could be let out and buttons moved over, which dresses could be altered enough to fit, and which ones couldn't. As I suffered through hours of these humiliating fittings, I could see my mother in all those mirrors. I wasn't the only one crawling with embarrassment.

She was the classic 50s stay-at-home mom, and I know my dad blamed her for not getting me to lose weight. She would retaliate by telling him I didn't get my fat from her side of the family (more on that later). I overheard many arguments between them about my weight. Knowing it was a source of a tremendous amount of friction in their marriage only added to my self-loathing.

Fast-forward to the hippie movement, which I thoroughly embraced in my high school and college years (1965 through 1974). It was during this time that I began to question all the things I had believed about being fat. It would prove to be a journey of many years to get from self-loathing to self-loving.

CHAPTER 2

# *The Current to Be Swum Against*

> It is clear from reading or watching television that public derision and condemnation of fat people is one of the few remaining sanctioned social prejudices in this nation freely allowed against any group based solely on appearance...
>
> —*Fitzgerald, Faith M.D., "The Problem of Obesity."* Annual Review of Medicine, *1981.*

I would love to report that things have really changed since 1981. If anything they have gotten worse. It felt necessary to start with a quote from a solid source because when I tell people I am openly hated by total strangers in public, they often don't believe me. Even many of my friends find this hard to believe and suspect I am exaggerating for effect (something I admittedly will do but only for humor's sake). As a matter of fact, I am feeling the need for even more backup before I tell some of my more personal experiences.

In an article dated 8/23/2012, Health Day reporter Amanda Gardner wrote:

> Many obese Americans say they face discrimination and stigma because of their weight a new Harris/Interactive poll found.... Much of this discrimination may still be socially acceptable: According to the poll, a majority of people (61%) do not consider negative remarks about a person's weight to be offensive.... That finding didn't surprise one medical expert. 'Although many deny it...there is enough scientific evidence that weight bias —which is more prevalent than race, sex, color, religious belief [bias]—is widespread and very resistant to change,' said Dr. Sarita Dhuper, Director of Pediatric Cardiology and Executive Director of the Live Light Live Right Pediatric Obesity Program at Brookdale University

> Hospital and Medical Center in New York City.

This next quote comes from an author you will find me citing a lot throughout this book, Glenn Gaesser. I'll hit you with all his considerable credentials at some point, but for now just trust me...this guy knows his stuff and does his homework!

In his book *Big Fat Lies: The Truth About Your Weight and Your Health*, Gaesser states:

> Fat people are routinely described as 'ugly,' 'disgusting,' 'sloppy,' and 'gross,' and characterized as 'weak willed,' 'self indulgent,' 'lacking in self respect,' 'emotionally disturbed,' and possibly 'sick.' Occasionally, the descriptions even veer into moral judgments as we denounce the fat person for failure to maintain his health for the sake of his family...or chide him for embarrassing his children in front of their friends.... If the attitudes of the society at large are not damning enough, surveys indicate that up to 88% of our healthcare professionals share one or all of these feelings. Indeed, the medical establishment has been largely responsible for our anti-fat crusade, giving it the imprimatur of science and thereby legitimizing it.... Medical, moral and esthetic

> condemnation of fat is now so pervasive in the United States that it ranks as a distinctive cultural trait. Fat phobia has become epidemic.
>
> In a poll of 1,000 women between the ages of 18 and 25, which ran in the February 1994 issue of Esquire, 54% stated they would rather be run over by a truck than be extremely fat. Two-thirds said they would rather be mean or stupid than fat. Is it any wonder that our young girls and women are experiencing an epidemic of anorexia and bulimia? Or that the same problems are beginning to afflict young men?

OK. I feel like I have enough outside support to tell a bit of my own experience without being accused of paranoia or exaggeration.

Sometimes when I am out in public, I get that prickly sensation at the back of my neck. I scan my surroundings to locate the source of my body's primal response to danger and invariably I find a woman. She is staring at me with such vehement loathing you would think I had not only murdered her firstborn but eaten him or her as well.

When I spot her, she doesn't look away in

embarrassment at being caught. Nope. She lifts her head a little higher, meets my eyes and glares even harder and nastier if possible. Why does this woman hate the sight of me, a complete stranger, so intensely? Why does she feel entitled to condemn me so proudly and openly?

It seems to me thin women who hate fat women take our being fat as some deep and very personal insult, maybe even a betrayal. We have openly challenged the FIB that keeps them chained to their diets and treadmills in fear of "letting themselves go."

I admit that I don't know what's behind their thinking as they openly stare at me with such disgust, and that's big of me because I really do believe I am on the right track. They have all drunk the FIB-flavored "Kool-Aid" and I suspect some of them hate me because clearly I have not, and they are jealous. I don't let society's fat rules rule me.

Do you think that sounds far-fetched? My mother gave me a lot of misinformation (some truly damaging but most of it simply hilarious), but she gave me a lot of quality wisdom, too. One of her best life lessons went like this, "If someone is trying to make your life miserable, you can bet they are jealous of you." I gotta tell you, in my experience she's been right 9.9 times out of 10.

So why would an officially society-stamped, approved-sized woman be jealous of big ol' me?

Well, while she leads her life of desperate deprivation, I am living a life of abundant sensual acceptance, no longer shackled by this society's expectations of what makes a beautiful woman.

I can't tell you how many women I've seen—fat and thin—obsessed with dieting and hating their perfectly beautiful bodies. It strikes me as a sad way to spend life's precious moments.

Now aside from staring at me in public with disgust and loathing, here's something else people, people who feel they are being kind and understanding by the way, feel free to do to me in public. Folks will come up to me, pat my arm in a show of commiseration, and say, "Inside every fat person there is a thin person crying to get out."

Really?!? Wow...you know...just... WOW!!! It is perfectly OK for any man, woman, or child to say those words anytime, anywhere. Would it be OK to say, "Inside every black person there's a white person crying to get out?" Not so much. Can you imagine the plenitude of poop that would hit the fan if someone said that? You would see headlines, national headlines, about that. But I think both statements are equal examples of ignorance and prejudice, both equally hurtful and insulting.

My guess is most fat people have someone inside crying Peter Finch's great line from *Network*: "I'm mad as hell and I'm not going to take it anymore" if they are harboring any inner stowaways at all.

So here's a message for all the haters out there from me. I would love to see you rethink this one. Let's call it consciousness-fattening instead of consciousness-raising. Expand your worldview to include those who are different from you, fatties among them. Yeah, I'm liking this idea. I'm not "morbidly obese," one of the most loathsome labels ever, BTW! I'm "expanded," literally and figuratively.

OK. It's one thing to call people on all this BS. The real trick is to stop believing it yourself! How did I get from self-loathing to self-loving? Read on....

CHAPTER 3

# *The TRUTH*

In most cases when people live under long-term oppression, they will eventually form a countermovement. There is just such a movement working to fight FIB. I have dubbed this resistance movement TRUTH, The Reality Underlying The Horsepoop. (Substitute "Hoax" or "Hooey" when in polite society.)

I was completely astonished to discover all the research papers and books that exist to support the conclusions I had come to through my own experiences. I want to share some of my take-aways from these writings.

So if you've stayed with me this far, you're probably wondering if so much of the stuff we are hammered with in the War on Obesity is indeed a pack of lies based on the false premise "Fat is Inherently Bad," what is really behind our nation's campaign against fatties? There's a saying that comes up time and time again when a mystery needs solving: "Follow the money."

Let me start with the book *Big Fat Lies: The Truth About Your Weight and Your Health* by Glenn A. Gaesser. I include a mere smattering of his credentials as promised lest you think I found some obscure lightweight who just happens to fall in line with my thinking.

> Glenn Gaesser is a professor of Exercise and Wellness in the School of Nutrition and Health Promotion, and is director of the Healthy Lifestyles Research Center, at Arizona State University. Professor Gaesser has had prior academic appointments at the University of Virginia and UCLA. He is a Fellow of the American College of Sports Medicine.
>
> Professor Gaesser's research focuses on the effects of exercise and diet on cardiovascular fitness and health and his work has been published in scientific journals, trade publications, newsletters and internet sites. He is the author or co-author of several books, including *Big Fat Lies: The Truth About Your Weight and Your Health* (Gurze, 2002) and *It's the Calories, Not the Carbs* (Trafford/Wheat Foods, 2004).

Professor Gaesser has given more than 250 invited regional and international presentations to a variety of professional, business, and lay audiences on the subjects of health, fitness and body weight, and is interviewed frequently by the media on these topics. He has had a number of television appearances, including *The Dr. Oz Show*, *Good Morning America*, ABC's *20/20*, *World News Tonight*, *NBC Nightly News*, CNN, *Dateline NBC*, and dozens of regional talk/news shows. In addition he has been a guest on more than 75 radio shows in North America and has been interviewed for stories on body weight, fitness and health for more than 100 newspapers and magazines throughout the world. In 1999 he received a public service award from the National Association of Anorexia Nervosa and Associated Disorders for his 'dedication to and promotion of health and rationality concerning body weight and fitness.'

Professor Gaesser was graduated Phi Beta Kappa from the University of California, Berkeley, where he also received his M.A. and Ph.D. degrees with a specialization in exercise physiology.

His book's introduction is a mind-blower all by itself. Not only does he follow the money trail to give an in-depth history of the birth and coming-of-age of the war on obesity, he cites study after study showing being fat is not at all the health menace it is touted as, and can often be more beneficial to your health than being thin. I'm not talking about studies done by "unheard of" people laboring in obscure corners of their fields. Gaesser presents evidence from well-respected professionals working at major universities and institutions published in the likes of *The New England Journal of Medicine* and *The Journal of the American Medical Association (JAMA).*

OK. Enough with the credentials and the accolades. Here comes just a smattering of the quotes I loved:

> There is a large and ever-growing body of scientific evidence, most of it still confined to professional journals, showing that fat may not be so bad and thin may not be so good. This is not to say that obesity is entirely benign or that body weight is unimportant to health. It's just that when you scrutinize all the relevant data it becomes apparent that the health risks of

> obesity, as well as the purported health benefits of weight loss, have been greatly exaggerated. Furthermore, the risks associated with weight loss have been under estimated.

Bam!! Oh, yeah!! Amen to that!!

Oops, I see that I strayed from my original intent to follow the money and see where the war on obesity started and how it grew to the ginormous absurdity blighting our society today.

Gaesser quotes, "Obesity, the Nutritional Spook," a 1971 article by George V. Mann, M.D., in *The American Journal of Public Health* for starters:

> The evil view of obesity has come from four places: the insurance industry, the medical moralizers (usually themselves thin), the drug industry and the docile, unquestioning nutritionists who are too often dupes of the faddists and hucksters.

Gaesser elaborates,

> A number of other culprits can be added to Dr. Mann's list, but two of them lead the pack: the fashion

> industry...and the fitness professionals, who have probably done more than any other group to make lean synonymous with healthy and fat with unhealthy. Collectively, all these forces have conspired to portray obesity in the most disparaging terms possible.

He cites the beginning of the War on Obesity as 1897(!) when the Metropolitan Life Insurance Company published their first Height-Weight Chart. He takes the reader on an odyssey through countless sources and studies showing how the insurance industry labored to get the medical profession on board and how the fashion industry helped. It makes for fascinating reading as the medical professionals weren't so easy to convince, given that it took a few decades or so. Their fat patients were generally far healthier and long-lived than their thin patients, you see.

But the insurance companies were unrelenting in preaching their anti-fat propaganda. Gaesser states,

> The efforts of Louis Dublin and his fellow life insurance medical directors were finally paying off. The turning point came in 1951. That was the year the campaign against obesity was taken up by the US Government and the

> medical establishment. Joining forces with the life insurance industry, the American Medical Association (AMA) and The United States Public Health Service embarked upon 'a nationwide effort... to stimulate interest anew in the problem of obesity and to spur positive action against it.' Fuelled by the combined forces of the medical community, the federal government, the life insurance industry and the world of fashion, the campaign for weight loss escalated at an exponential rate of growth, and the media delivered the message.

This timing holds special significance for me as I was born in 1951. I got to experience my "exponential rate of growth" right along with the war on obesity's. Yep, I am well known for my impeccable timing.

Gaesser continues,

> In 1985 a US government sponsored conference on 'The Health Implications of Obesity,' under the aegis of the NIH, may even have taken the battle to a new level of intensity. Though the panel's scientists issued a rather clinical and familiar sounding statement about how 'obesity, defined as

excessive storage of energy in the form of fat, has adverse effects on health and longevity' the story got sensationalized by such newspaper headlines as 'Obesity is 'Killer Disease' Affecting 34 Million Americans, NIH Reports' and 'Panel Finds Obesity a Major US Killer.' The fact that experts at the conference presented a large amount of data questioning the prevailing assumptions about weight, health and longevity did not find its way into the popular press nor was that material reflected in the panel's 'consensus' statement.... Although anti-obesity warriors are convinced, and have done a good job convincing us, that weight loss itself improves health and lengthens life, there are absolutely no studies that unequivocally show this to be true. In fact, many studies indicate that voluntary weight loss may compromise health and increase risk for premature death.... Of all our convictions about health, 'Thinner is Healthier' has no rival when it comes to the gap between belief and evidence. There is a lot of evidence that suggests the opposite, evidence that for the most part has gone unheeded, never having made

> the leap from medical journals into the popular press."

How much do I love and adore this guy?! His book is a MUST READ, really. Not only does he do an amazing job citing research and data dating from the 1800s to today (even quoting Hippocrates), he also offers a nice fitness plan that seems eminently sensible and "doable" to me (get the book!!). He has utterly convinced me that fitness is a must for my health, and his program is not crazy or impossible or even unpleasant to contemplate...I am in!

Ah, I seem to have veered a micro-tad off following that money trail once again. It's pretty obvious when you think about it. The diet industry reaps $50 billion +/- a year in America. One of the beauties of Gaesser's book is the impressive investigative job he does following the money from the insurance industry to the health professionals in league with the diet industry to the fitness industry. He even shows how government policy has been shaped to keep money flowing in the desired directions. The War on Obesity is a tribute to capitalism at its nasty, greedy worst. The uber-FIB: It damages your health and your psyche while it takes your money, promising the exact opposite: a happier, healthier you.

Gaesser again:

...The more than $30 billion a year Americans shelled out in the 1990s is now estimated to be close to $50 billion per year despite the less-than-stellar results.... Dieting almost always promotes the very thing it is supposed to cure: obesity.

CHAPTER 4

# *FIB²s*

This chapter is all about challenging $FIB^2$s. What is a $FIB^2$ you might ask? It means FIB squared and references a math term for a number multiplied by itself. For example: 4 is $2^2$ (2x2). So a $FIB^2$ is any fib that comes from the primal concept Fat Is Bad. This may not be a perfect analogy, but I like it and I'm sticking with it.

Again, an example:

If "Fat Is Bad" = FIB   Then,
"You won't live as long if you are fat." = $FIB^2$

Or,

"Fat people are lazy." Or,
"Fat people are gluttons."

That list can go on and on. They are all $FIB^2$s. I think it's time to challenge some of this BS!

One FIB[2] I have understandably given a lot of thought to is, "Being fat will shorten your life." You hear that everywhere. I heard it from my parents my whole life, and from most of my doctors and most of my friends. Well, I think some key words got left out. Here's my take on it:

Being fat IN AMERICA could definitely shorten your life.

Yep. After living my life fat from birth to the present moment, I truly believe in that statement. As already stated, this country has openly, sanctimoniously, and proudly declared war on fat.

Years ago when America declared war on smokers, I had one main and selfish thought: I hoped the smokers would fight back long and hard. They took the major heat off fatties for a while, but I knew once they fell, the heat would be back on us with laser intensity. It was a no-brainer.

It bears repeating that in America it has always been okay to openly stare and glare at fat people, to mock us. Fat jokes are okay to tell anywhere, anytime. Political correctness has put many subjects off-limits in 'polite society'—fat is not one of them. Living in a country where you are bombarded with officially sanctioned anti-fat sentiments everywhere you turn is extremely stressful... and people...stress kills!!

You know by now how I love quotes. I think it comes from all the years of watching *Reading*

*Rainbow* with my kids. "You don't have to take my word for it."

> At a National Institute of Health (NIH) conference on obesity it was acknowledged that obesity creates an enormous psychological burden. In terms of suffering, this burden may be the greatest adverse effect of obesity, — Glenn Gaesser.

Gaesser also states researchers have concluded, "Stress itself may cause the expansion of bad body fat. Other health consequences in the stressed group included high blood pressure, elevated blood fats, and heart disease."

Anyway, there are a gazillion studies out there saying stress kills. And people, I repeat, being fat in America can be very stressful!

While working on this chapter, I got to wondering if there were any countries where fat was enthusiastically embraced. Here's the good news: There are countries on this planet that not only think fat is ok, they think it is fabulous! And since I was addressing the longevity FIB$^2$, I started wondering... You thought I'd lost the thread didn't you? I googled some of these countries and got the statistics on their Female Average Life Expectancy (FALE).

So how do female fatties fare in terms of

longevity in some countries where fat is where it's at?

Samoa FALE – 76 years

Kuwait FALE – 80 years

Fiji FALE – 72 years

Jamaica FALE – 78 years

Tahiti FALE – 78.6 years

And drum roll, please. On Nauru, where according to statistics the world's most obese people live, FALE is 76.

I always knew there was a reason tropical islands beckoned to me. The FALE in America is 81. I have to tell you I would gladly trade 2.4 years of life in a country that hates me to go live in Tahiti and croak at 78.6. Yep, if the war on fat is won, I definitely want to be exiled to Tahiti!

A major FIB[2] I have questioned aggressively and resented for years is that fatties are such an egregious burden on our healthcare system.

That FIB[2] is the martial drumbeat of the war on fat in my opinion. If you want to stir up anger and resentment in an American and get him on board with your cause, just tell him your target is hurting his pocketbook.

Now I'm not saying fat folks don't have an impact on our healthcare system. As previously stated, I would say it is the stress of being fat in America, courteously provided by FIB believers on a daily basis, that is causing their health woes. But that's not even the point I want to make about this particular FIB².

One of my daughters is a first-degree black belt in kung fu. She would probably be a third degree or higher by now, but she suffered a mishap a few years ago that ended her kung fu career. She was doing one of those amazing flying kick jumps and landed wrong. Her ACL was torn so severely it required replacement with a donor's ACL and lots of titanium pins.

I went with her to every doctor and physical therapist visit pre- and postsurgery. What I saw got me pondering.

All of these waiting rooms were full of young, thin patients with a smattering of older folks scattered among them. I was usually the only fatty there, and I wasn't a patient.

So my question is, What kind of a burden do sports and fitness injuries place on our healthcare system? Once again I turned to Google (God I love computers!) and came up with some eye-opening info.

The Centers for Disease Control (CDC) did a study in June 2002 titled, "CDC Injury Research Agenda."

Here are some of the juicy facts they gathered on SER (sports, exercise, and recreation) injuries way back then. In the ensuing twelve years, I can only imagine these figures have probably gone up.

"More than 10,000 people receive treatment in the nation's emergency departments (ED) each day for injuries sustained in SER activities."

Wow—just—wow. Do you think 10,000 fatties hit the EDs in this country *every day*? I feel like I could rest my case on that little factoid alone, but this report from the CDC is the gift that just keeps on giving. Buckle your seatbelts people who think fatties are the big villains overburdening the healthcare system...you're in for the proverbial bumpy ride:

> In 1999, Americans made an estimated 1.5 million ED visits for injuries sustained while playing basketball, baseball, softball, football, or soccer.
>
> Children younger than 15 account for... about 40% of all SER-related ED visits.
>
> Adolescents and young adults under age 25...experience almost one third of all SER-related injuries.
>
> The population of older adults is increasing and little is known about their injury risk during participation in SER. In 1996, emergency departments treated more than 53,000 SER-related injuries among people 65 and older, a 54% increase from 1990.

> Approximately 73,000 ED visits annually are related to participation in equestrian activities alone, and many thousands of people are injured each year while using personal recreational vehicles.
>
> Approximately 81 million people ride bicycles, and each year, more than 600,000 visit the ED for bicycle-related injuries.
>
> A 1994 survey reported that 20% of adults (38 million) ride bicycles outdoors and 73% (138 million) walked for exercise in the 30 days before the survey. During this time period, 1% to 1.5% reported that they were injured while doing these activities.

OK, folks. I did the math on that one. Just using the lowball one percent, that works out to 380,000 cyclists and 1,380,000 walkers injured in a thirty-day period.

Here are what I can only call some stunning facts from this same CDC report on ACL injuries—my daughter's burden on the healthcare system.

> In the U.S., anterior cruciate ligament (ACL) knee injuries are usually sports related, and the vast majority occur in active, healthy 15- to 24-year olds (my daughter). ACL rupture can

> be debilitating in the short term, preventing continued physical activity. (Yep, my daughter.) The cost of ACL reconstruction alone, *not including evaluation or rehabilitation* (my italics), is just under *$1 billion per year* (my italics) in the U.S.

This CDC report is so mind-blowing. It is amazing to see something I have suspected for years backed up by such eye-opening statistics. Wouldn't it be nice if a few minds opened as well? But wait. I saved the best for last.

> SER injuries...place a large burden on the healthcare system for both initial care and rehabilitation. They also result in costs related to lost productivity and other factors. Despite the large number of ED visits for these injuries, most medically treated SER-related injuries are treated by healthcare providers outside of the emergency setting, indicating that *the magnitude of the problem is much greater than ED statistics suggest* (my italics).

BAM!!! Take that all you idiots out there beating the "Fatties overburden the healthcare system" drum! So what do you think, you sanctimonious morons: Should there be a War on Fitness based on the staggering burden *IT places on the health-care system?*

Don't demonize 'FAT' if you aren't going to demonize 'FIT'... that's all I'm saying.

And while I am bandying about the words fat and fit, this is as good a place as any to ask, Can you be fat and fit? (Wait a minute. Would that make you a double burden on the healthcare system?)

OK, that one is too convoluted for me so let's just stick with the question. Can you be fit and fat? You bet your sweet "Baby Got Back" booty you can!

Here are some great excerpts from an article I found at *Fitness Magazine* online by Peg Rosen titled "Can you be Fat but Fit?"

> There are two large women who've been in boot camp with me for years. They almost never miss a class and never take it easy. Yet as I've lunged, squatted, and planked alongside them nearly daily, I'm ashamed to admit that one question has occasionally bounced around my brain: With all that exercise, after all this time, why aren't these women in better shape?
>
> Then came the 2012 Olympic Games. The world was poised to witness its most formidable female athletes lock horns in London. And what did we hear? Slams against Australian swimmer Leisel

> Jones, declaring the eight-time medalist fat and thus unfit to represent her country; cheap shots about muffin tops and saddlebags on the British women's beach volleyball team; and tweets about British swimmer Rebecca Adlington's physique that became so vicious, she dropped off Twitter altogether. "These women made it to the Olympics, for God's sake. How unfit could they be?" I found myself ranting at the TV.
>
> Then I thought, sheepishly, about the women at boot camp. It became clear to me that the knee-jerk connection I and apparently others might make between how much a person weighs and how physically fit and healthy she is needed some serious reevaluation.

If you want to be fit, you have to give that aforementioned booty at least twenty minutes of exercise three days a week. That's the minimum requirement. I cannot tell you the myriad places that advice shows up.

While researching this book, I became utterly convinced I need to get into an exercise program, especially since I retired a year ago from a very physical job and have been duffing it ever since. So 2014 has seen me engaging in a love-hate relationship with my treadmill. I don't know if I will succeed in getting exercise into my daily routine, but I am really going to give it a try.

Here are some more interesting tidbits on FIB²'s relating to health. Let's stay with Peg Rosen's *Fitness Magazine* article for a minute.

> Recent research suggests that being overweight or even obese may not, in and of itself, be the health threat we think it is. A 2012 study from the National Cancer Institute found that moderately obese people actually lived about 3.1 years longer than normal-weight women and men. Another study, published in the *European Heart Journal,* showed that when obese people are metabolically healthy—which means blood pressure, cholesterol, blood sugar and other indicators fall within a healthy range—they are at no greater risk of dying from heart disease or cancer than those who are of normal weight.

And once again I am going to dip into Glenn Gaesser's book, *Big Fat Lies: The Truth About Your Weight and Your Health.* He is totally my hero, totally.

> Men and women medically classified as 'overweight' or 'obese' have lower

> risks of lung cancer (both smokers and nonsmokers) and osteoporosis than men and women who are either thin or of average weight.
>
> The 'thinner is better' studies frequently cited by healthcare professionals are far outnumbered by studies showing that—aside from the very extremes—body weight is fairly unrelated to health status and death rates or that weights above those recommended by the height-weight tables are actually better for health and longevity.
>
> If obesity is a killer disease, as the chairman of the obesity conference told newspaper reporters in 1985, and one that affects tens of millions of Americans, then we might reasonably expect it to be implicated in atherosclerosis, or clogged arteries, which is the number one killer in America. Not only do most data fail to support that hypothesis, but few of the available data support any of the numerous hypotheses about overweight as a primary cause of any of the major diseases for which it is routinely blamed (with the exception of osteoarthritis).

Here's a doozy from Gaesser:

> ...Former Surgeon General C. Everett Koop, in launching his 'Shape Up America' campaign (see CDC report on SER injuries I think to myself sarcastically)...claimed that obesity kills more than 300,000 Americans every year.
>
> Subsequently, this statistic has surfaced repeatedly in newspapers, magazines, television, and radio broadcasts and in many scientific journals—each time proclaiming obesity the second leading preventable cause of death (next to smoking) in the United States.... What surprises me, given the gravity of the statistic, is that no one seems to have bothered to verify it.

Yep, good ole Glenn, a man I have come to worship, goes on for pages shooting down that 300,000 claim and backing himself up all the way with facts. Seriously, people, have I mentioned his book is a *must read*?

Let's close this chapter with another major FIB². Dieting is good for you. Really?... is it? Once again I am going to quote some authorities on the subject.

First, a refresher quote: Remember follow the money?

Gaesser states, "The 120 million people who are trying to lose or maintain weight via reduced calorie intake have turned dieting into a 30 billion dollar plus industry (with some estimates much higher than that)."

Yes indeedy. A lot of folks have a vested interest in keeping FIB alive and well. Whether any of it is true or not...they definitely want us dieting.

But here's a shocker....

> "Until we have better data about the risks of being overweight and the benefits and risks of trying to lose weight, we should remember that the cure for obesity may be worse than the condition." —Jerome P. Kassirer, M.D., and Marcia Angell, M.D.; Editors, *The New England Journal of Medicine*, January 1, 1998.

Hmm. I didn't see any headlines on that. Did you?

Want to hear more? Of course you do. I know I did.

"Body fat is not lethal, but the effort to get rid of it can be," says Gaesser.

Now that would have made an excellent headline and a fantastic sound bite. But nobody's beating us over the head with that one are they? Follow the money.

> ...The health risks of dieting have largely been ignored. Dieting, particularly the yo-yo dieting that is very much the norm for millions of women,

> may increase the risk for a number of diseases, including cardiovascular disease, type 2 diabetes, osteoporosis, and certain cancers. Even mental function may be affected. (also from Gaesser)

I'm not too sure this horse (FIB²—Dieting is a good thing) is dead so I feel the need to beat it with Glenn Gaesser's hammer one more time. You can tell I'm enjoying this, right? I mean I am laughing out loud while I type most of these quotes:

> By 1966 researchers had made such a powerful case concerning the hazards of yo-yoing that the U.S. Government itself spoke out, in the form of a 77 page report on 'Obesity and Health'... Nine experts in the field of health and nutrition used the report as a forum to warn the public that '...the frequent weight gains and losses indulged in by many obese patients...may be actually more harmful than maintenance of a steady weight at a high level.'

Huh? 1966 people! I yo-yo'd from the 1960s to the 1990s, and I never saw hide nor hair of that report anywhere. I yo-yo'd so much I probably spontaneously sprouted a tramp stamp that says "Duncan." I'll bet those nine experts and all seventy-seven pages of that report are buried together in a very deep hole somewhere, maybe keeping Jimmy Hoffa company.

OK, I'm almost done, I promise. One more quote from my hero (you know his name; buy his book!):

> Eating disorders, particularly bulimia, are another possible consequence of our national obsession with thinness and the chronic dieting it promotes. Many experts today view dieting as an intermediate stage between normal eating and eating disorders.

How about that? Dieting as a "gateway drug" to eating disorders...huh. Who'd a thunk it?

So there are a lot of the reasons, not all—I could have gone on for many more pages, trust me—why I absolutely do not believe FIB in general and the myriad FIB$^2$s in particular.

I realize the fact that I don't choose to believe all this FIB propaganda doesn't mean it might not have some validity. No one has proved any of it to my satisfaction, though. Frankly, even if they could I don't think I would choose constant deprivation, obsessive thinking about food, and all the attendant misery dieting caused me. It's not the life I want. My life as a self-loving fatty is a mostly joyous and always fulfilled one.

CHAPTER 5

# *The Planet Fat*

My kids and I are huge sci-fi fans. The thought of space travel and life on other planets is exciting and seductive for us. But I have always told them they don't need to look to space for countless fascinating life-forms because they are already here on this amazing planet.

Greetings, earthlings. I am from the planet Fat. I come in peace and mean you no harm.

Somewhere along my seemingly endless cycles of losing weight only to gain it all back and then some (the infamous and, as previously mentioned, very unhealthy yo-yo dieting), I began to feel it just didn't make sense. Why was it so friggen hard to lose the weight in the first place but so very easy to gain it all back with a few extra new pounds tacked on as my bonus prize?

I began to suspect I was simply meant to

be fat. I was born that way and it was my natural body type. I didn't share this suspicion with anyone because I figured they would just see it as my excuse. How big an aha! moment do you think I had when the "fat gene" was discovered?

My father had tipped the scales at 300+ pounds until his college fraternity brothers "forced" (his word) him to lose the weight. He never went into the details of how they managed it, but he watched his weight (read... restricted his diet severely) for the rest of his life.

Starting around the time I was age 6 or so, my dad would have a serious talk with me once or twice a year about my weight. He would paint a very grim picture of what my future held if I failed to thin down. He spoke with kindness and concern, but the first few talks ended with me in tears. Dad was no doubt hoping they were a sign the message had hit home and the fearful picture of my doomed future as a fatty was making me cry. But I was crying because the message I was getting was that he couldn't love me fat; I was a disappointment and an embarrassment. As the lectures kept coming year after year all the way through high school and beyond (a very sad father-daughter tradition), I learned to bear them with a small smile while my heart broke and my self-image took another blow.

Yep, my take-away from Dad's talks and Mom's endless attempts to put me on every diet she ever heard of was that my being fat was a never-ending source of shame for them. They were buying into society's judgment that "Fat Is Bad" big-time. My fat symbolized their failure as parents. Society reinforced that belief at every turn, right down to their friends who commiserated with them about my weight "problem." How do I know that ever happened, you ask? They did it right in front of me all the time.

My being fat became a morbidly obese sore spot in their marriage as the years passed. They argued about it in front of me, and I often overheard them arguing about it "in private." Dad blamed Mom for not monitoring my diet properly (though she did). Mom would hurl back, "She didn't get it from *my* side of the family!" (Whoa... did my mother actually discover the fat gene back in the 1950s?) And they both blamed me for not trying hard enough.

I don't tell you this as a sympathy ploy. I tell you this to demonstrate how insidious and destructive buying into our society's *opinion,* not a fact mind you, can be. Believing FIB tainted my childhood and my parents' marriage. It drained pleasure from their lives until the day they died and from mine as well until I finally saw FIB for what it is, a monstrous lie.

But enough about me for the moment. Here are some of the more scintillating bits of info from

Gaesser I came across on the genetics of fat.

> The number of fat cells can range from around 20 billion in a lean person to 100 billion or more in a very fat person…. The reason for the wide variation…is not entirely understood, but appears to be largely a matter of genes. The genetic component of our fat makeup is, so far as we know, unalterable.
>
> Anyone who feels overly heavy could follow the recommendation to 'be active and eat less fat' and find his or her way to a healthier weight…but there is a catch. The number of fat cells won't diminish, and the size of a fat cell can only get so low, and that's it. While some people may have lower set points for the amount of fat in each cell, for each of us there is some limit, which no amount of lifestyle is going to be able to change.
>
> Current medical and scientific guidelines and the health practitioners and doctors who issue them do not take into account individual variations in set point. They put an overweight label on millions of fat people whose fat cells are numerous but happen to be at a "healthy" size, and they give a false

> sense of security to millions of thin and average weight people with relatively few fat cells all of which may be bursting at the seams thanks to a daily regimen of too much junk food and too little exercise.

Here are some excerpts I found fascinating from an article dated 1/10/2013 titled "'Fat Genes' Determine Obesity, UCLA Study Says, In Addition to Diet and Exercise," by Kathleen Miles on *The Huffington Post*:

> While diet and exercise are still large factors in obesity, the degree to which one gains weight from a high-fat diet is largely determined by genetics, according to researchers.
>
> In the study, funded by the National Institute of Health and appearing in the print version of the journal Cell Metabolism, UCLA researchers gave more than 100 genetic strains of mice a normal diet for 8 weeks, followed by a high-fat, high-sugar diet for another 8 weeks.
>
> Even though the mice were eating the exact same diets, their weight gain varied greatly. The high-fat diet caused no change in body fat percentage for some mice while others' body fat percentages *increased by a whopping*

> *600 percent*. (My italics!!)
>
> 'We've all seen those people who eat a lot and don't gain weight...' (cruelly, I was married to one of them - author comment) principal investigator Dr. Jake Lusis, a professor of Medicine and Human Genetics and of Microbiology, Immunology and Molecular Genetics at the Geffen School of Medicine told *The Huffington Post*. 'It isn't just all about how much we eat. Genes had a huge effect.'

Here are some snippets from an article that appeared in the Health and Family section of *Time* dated 7/19/2013, titled "New Genes ID'd in Obesity: How much of Weight is Genetic?" by Alexandria Sifferlin.

> In two separate papers published in The Journal of Science and in the Journal of Clinical Investigation (JCI), researchers describe new genetic factors that could explain weight gain in some people.
>
> Genome-wide association studies, which compare genetic makeups of obese individuals to those of normal weight, are making it easier to flesh out important genetic factors contributing to weight, and researchers at the Harvard School of Public Health say that

> to date these studies have identified over 30 candidate genes on 12 chromosomes associated with body mass index.

Ok. If you haven't gotten the point by now,...right?

So to sum up:

I was born plump and have always been fat. After years of yo-yo dieting through my teens and twenties, I finally came to the conclusion that I was born to be big. Now I find out I am right up there with the folks with five times the amount of fat cells as thin folks and the mice whose body fat percentages increased 600% on the same diet as their lean counterparts. What the hell.

It is a hoot to see my suspicions borne out by science. Feels like a victory to me. Shall I say, tastes sweet? Oh, yeah!!

CHAPTER 6

# *The Choice—To BElieve or Not To BElieve*

So realizing you are trapped in FIB is just the beginning. Fighting your way out of it can be a struggle of epic proportions.

I don't remember when I first started thinking or suspecting that FIB was a big crock. Events that made me stop and go "Huh?" stand out in my mind, but I can't place them chronologically.

As a child I was so miserable believing in FIB the seeds to my liberation were undoubtedly sown in that soil. I can remember vehemently thinking to myself so many times, "How can things be so unfair?" Maybe that mantra was the start of my journey to the realization that I didn't have to believe everything society was pushing as truth.

One of the most vivid "HUH?" moments I will never forget started with channel surfing. I'm not a big talk show fan in general, but a *Sally Jessy Raphael Show* years ago made me stop clicking my remote.

There was a fat lady on stage and the audience was in full attack mode, I kid you not. They were really whipped up by the time I tuned in so I can only assume it had been going on for a while.

A thin woman, voice charged with loathing, asked, "Do you really expect me to believe you don't eat any more food than I do?" (Remember those mice, people?) as the audience hooted and jeered. The fat lady tried to answer, but the audience abuse continued.

Another person rudely asked, "How do *you people* have sex anyway?" with plenty of disgust spinning that question, I kid you not. The fat lady answered, "The same way you do." with as much attitude as she dared muster...and it wasn't much.

What did Sally Jessy Raphael do? How did she respond in a situation where a vicious audience was attacking her guest? Did she challenge the lynch mob? Call them out in any way?

Nope. She turned to the fat lady and said critically, "I have to say, you do sound a bit defensive."

Wow. Like I said...one of the biggest "HUH?" moments of my life.

FIB is everywhere in our lives, nowhere

more obvious and insidious than in the media. FIB pervades TV from sitcoms to reality shows. (If beings from another planet ever visit and happen to see an episode of *The Biggest Loser*, they'll think we are a society of barbaric torturers.) It's in our movies, our literature (fiction and nonfiction), our magazines, on the radio, on the Internet. FIB spawned its own multimillion (hell, multibillion dollar probably) industry with diet pills, diet doctors, diet books, diet gurus, fitness experts ad nauseam, heavy on the nauseam.

There are way too many prejudices in this world to list them here. This book is devoted to just one of them, but I am not suggesting that being prejudiced against fat people is the worst one. I am simply writing about the prejudice that affected my life for years because I believed it and still affects my life today because others believe it.

***Digression Alert***

Remember the ditty "Big Girls Don't Cry"? Well fat girls don't fly—at least without major difficulties, and that brings up an important point.

Liberating yourself from FIB doesn't mean you won't still be affected by it, thanks to its faithful adherents. You will be turned down for jobs because you are fat. I was many times and told so right to my face in the days before you could sue for discrimination.

Suing may prove to be a step forward in the long term, but short term it has mainly just driven some FIB prejudice underground. It is still alive and well out there just waiting to bite you in your splendid booty. You will not get jobs for which you are well qualified. Studies show fat people are less likely to be promoted once they do find a job and are often paid less than their thin co-workers for doing the same job. I could go on and on about the negative impacts society's belief in FIB can have on a fatty's life.

I know I already said this, but it's worth repeating. There are way too many prejudices out there. More than enough for everyone to be hit one way or another. I mean even beautiful blondes are dumb, right?

I can claim to be the victim of prejudice on at least four counts myself:

- FIB'ism
- Sexism
- Ageism
- Anti-Semitism

Like I said, there's plenty of nasty "isms" out there.

What I really try to be careful about is not saying something is coming from prejudice when it may not be.

OK, after all that I am back to fat girls flying. A while back there was a hoo-ha about some airlines deciding to charge oversize people for two seats. Some members of the fat community were pissed off and attacked the airlines for the decision claiming discrimination.

I really didn't follow it too closely and I don't know where it stands today because I thought the airlines were right. I didn't take it personally as an attack on fat. It's just business, in my opinion.

If you are taking up more than one seat, then you need to pay for two. It isn't fair for you to encroach on another passenger's space, and it isn't fair to expect the airline to "comp" you an extra seat. If you need more space, you need to pay for it.

My point is even once a person achieves a healthy attitude about him- or herself, it doesn't mean their life will be free from the repercussions of prejudice. I try not to see FIB around every corner, that's all. I don't deny it is pervasive, but I don't believe it accounts for every difficulty I might face.

Wow. Ok, all that writing and I still haven't told you how I went from self-loathing to self-loving.

Well, as I said, even as a child I knew it wasn't a good thing to be hating myself. It sounds pretty basic, but it is really important to know that, maybe even the first step to overcoming it.

In *Annie Hall* Woody Allen steals a great Groucho Marx quip and says something like,

"I wouldn't want to belong to any club that would accept me as a member." That really says it all, doesn't it? What's wrong with him if he's interested in me? What's wrong with that person if he or she wants to be my friend? Ugh, really self-defeating, poisonous thinking, right?

So the boring part of my journey to self-esteem was just lecturing myself internally on pretty much a daily basis. It's where my manifesto was born. If you listen to an idea long enough, you just might begin to believe it.

Well, my lecture program may have been slowly convincing me I was actually deserving of admiration, respect, and even love, but in my early twenties, I was still extremely insecure about my body. So I decided some shock therapy was what I needed next.

I got my BA in ceramics and sculpture from Bennington College in Vermont. After graduating I got a job as a ceramic prof's assistant at Skidmore College. The job was a blast, but the pay wasn't.

I decided to take a giant step in liberating myself from FIB's curse on my body image and make some money while doing so. No, I did not take up the world's oldest profession. I signed up to do nude modeling for the drawing classes at the college.

Fat is more interesting and challenging to draw, and I quickly became a much called upon model. I was just quaking inside the first time I stood nude before a class. But each time I disrobed and let a room full of my peers stare intently at my naked body for hours on end, I could feel FIB losing its grip on me.

There's a funny sidebar to this story, and in the interests of making a short story long I'm going to tell it. As I said, I was very into ceramics at the time and there happened to be a professional potter living in the area whose work I greatly admired. I was trying to work up the nerve to go out to his studio and meet him. I needed courage not because I was fat and feared his judgment, but because I was worried he might turn out to be an asshole. It sucks when someone you admire turns out to be a jerk upon closer inspection.

Anyway, my nude modeling was going so well I decided to increase that source of income. I headed off campus to a community arts center and got modeling gigs there as well.

One evening as I was putting my robe on to take a break, one of the artists approached me. He told me he thought I was an amazing model and was wondering if I would consider coming to model privately for him at his studio. Guess who!

Yep, it was my idol. To this day I laugh out loud when I remember meeting him under those circumstances. He was not a jerk, and it was the start of a nice friendship.

Other than nude modeling and constant pep talks to myself, reading helped me a lot. I don't mean self-help books. I came across a lot of helpful stuff just reading in general, everything from biographies to blogs, fiction and nonfiction, poetry, history, philosophy. I am what they call an avid reader.

I like to collect my favorite quotes from things I read. Here are a few that definitely helped me on my way to self-esteem:

From Eleanor Roosevelt (hands down our greatest First Lady ever):

> You can often change your circumstances by changing your attitude.
>
> Life is what you make it. Always has been, always will be.
>
> No one can make you feel inferior without your consent.
>
> When you adopt the standards and the values of someone else…you surrender your own integrity. You become, to the extent of your surrender, less of a human being.
>
> In the long run we shape our lives and we shape ourselves. The process never ends until we die and the choices we make are ultimately our own responsibility.

From Ralph Waldo Emerson:

> To be yourself in a world that is constantly trying to make you something else is the greatest accomplishment.

And a very fun and really true one from Steven Winterburn (widely attributed to William Gibson who disavows it and refers folks to Winterburn's Twitter page):

> Before you diagnose yourself with depression or low self-esteem, first make sure that you are not, in fact, just surrounding yourself with assholes.

OK. I'm sure you get the proverbial drift...words not only to live by but to change by. We may indeed be what we eat, but we are absolutely what we believe!

I suppose I need to say something about FIB and my sex life. It is 2014 after all. Since my children will likely read this book at some point, I'll do the nitty without the gritty.

I can't say how deeply FIB has affected my relationships with the opposite sex. While I fully embraced and willingly participated in the Hippie culture in almost every way, I was an observer only of the free love part. Hmmm. That reads naughtier than I intend it. I was a non-participant, not a voyeur! I did get lots of offers back then, so it wasn't for lack of opportunity.

By my late teens I was really working hard to overcome my self-loathing, but the risk of having my naked body mocked or scorned by a sex partner was more than I was willing to take. I was afraid one bad episode in the boudoir would set back my journey to self-love (hmm, that sounds a bit naughty in this context, too, but you all know what I mean) years, if not derail it permanently.

I often joke that I am probably the only person on the planet born in 1951 who emerged from the free-Love generation AND graduated Bennington College a virgin!

I was 25 before I had the guts to go to bed with a man, and luckily for me he was a perfect gentleman. I think I was still fragile enough about my body image that he could have done some real damage if he had been a jerk in any way. Even during our "breakup" with all the attendant pyrotechnics he never once criticized me for being too fat or undesirable. They do say good things come to those who wait. Well the universe smiled and sent me a mensch!

Now FIB can affect your mind in some more subtle ways as well as the obvious—or at least it does mine. I'll tell you the story of my last boyfriend as an example. In fact, my OCD requires the symmetry...you get it...first boyfriend story → last boyfriend story.

There was an absolutely gorgeous guy, I mean

put him on the cover of *Esquire*-gorgeous—who started making deliveries to my workplace. I am a big flirt, but you have to be careful in this day and age of political correctness, when you can get sued for sexual harassment for a pat on the shoulder. So I flat out asked him if innocent flirtations would offend him. He laughed and encouraged me to flirt all I liked as long as he could flirt back.

Thus began many fun flirtations between him and me. I would come home and share these exchanges with my daughters. After hearing only a couple of these stories, my eldest said, "Mom, he's not flirting with you. He means it." I laughed in her face and said, "Honey, he's years younger than I (22 to be exact) and drop-dead gorgeous. There is no way he means it. We're just having fun."

Now you are thinking. Ah-hah! She says she's overcome her fat hang-ups about her body but she hasn't really.

Well, here's where it gets tricky. I didn't think he was seriously interested in me because ***I*** believed in FIB. I was assuming he couldn't be serious because *he* believed in FIB.

I mean let's face reality here. Most guys in this country subscribe to FIB. I just figured he was one of the majority, happy to flirt with some fat woman he found clever and amusing but not wanting to get her into the bedroom for real.

This flirtation went on for months, and every

time I reported an incident, my daughter would look at me like I was twenty kinds of stupid, shake her head, and repeat, "Mom, he's not kidding with you."

So one day after a major flirt-a-thon, I looked him right in the eye and asked, "We're just having fun here, right? I mean none of this is serious is it?" He looked right back in my eyes and said, "I don't know about you, but I mean every word of it."

What happened after that isn't subject matter for this book. To say I have yet to live this down with my daughter is putting it mildly. She's never going to let me forget it!

Lesson learned: If not believing FIB personally is step one, allowing yourself to believe there are others who don't believe FIB is step two.

When I finally unlocked the door behind which my self-esteem was imprisoned, the escaping positive thinking burst out like a tidal wave, a veritable tsunami of self-approval. The pendulum swung from self-loathing to self-love so violently it got stuck there and has yet to move back to a sane position of being comfortably satisfied with myself. In fact, I would even be willing to apply the utterly putrescent term "morbidly obese" to my ego. I do think it may be a bit out of control and could use a diet of less saturated pride and more high fiber humility.

The friends who manage to put up with me will all testify that nobody loves me more than I do. But I am a hell of a lot more fun than the self-loather of old. And hey, a girl's gotta make up for lost time, right?

CHAPTER 7

# The Home Stretch

Okay. You remember way back in my introduction I told you I was a master at making a short story long? I'm almost done, truly. In my defense, here is the short story:

- » I was born, and have always been, fat.
- » For most of my first three decades I believed FIB and had majorly low self-esteem.
- » I stopped believing FIB and lived happily (as anyone can in this day and age) ever after.

See? I can do it, but how much fun is that to read? So I think all that is left before I present my manifesto is to tell you a bit about my happily ever after.

I believe I need to pick up my personal narrative at the point where I had finally summoned up enough self-confidence to have a lover. While I was with that first boyfriend, I actually met my husband-to-be and that's the story I want to tell you now.

My future mate ran a family business in a town in New York just over the border from Bennington, Vermont. It was a huge, sprawling antique store. I had driven by it countless times during my college years and had always thought it amazingly intriguing as I cruised past on my way to wherever. I would always think, next time I have *got* to check that place out, but I never did.

Flash forward three or four years after my graduation from Bennington. I was living in the area again and with my aforementioned "first love." A friend had brought her latest beau up for a weekend visit. He happened to mention he was having no luck finding a certain antique lamp—he had been looking for ages and wondered if there were any good places around to go antiquing. That seductive antique store I had been meaning to check out for years came immediately to mind and off we went.

The store was insanely huge...three floors packed with everything imaginable. The owner approached us and my friend's boyfriend inquired about his elusive lamp. The owner gestured toward an area further back in the store and said all the lamps were there. (I will be refraining from description and calling my husband "the owner" because that is all I really thought of him as during this visit.)

Our guys headed for the lamps, and my friend and I headed for the antique clothes. The owner stuck to us and in spite of repeated avowals that we were just looking, he wouldn't leave us alone. Finally, we were forced to insist that he allow us to browse in peace while he waited on the guy who actually wanted to buy something.

He reluctantly left us and I remember turning to my friend and observing he must have been hitting on her. (I assumed he was interested in her because she was a trim little blonde. While I was accepting myself by then, I still knew nine out of ten guys in our society would choose her over me. That old saying about "assume making an ass of you and me" was at least half true that day.) We both laughed and promptly forgot all about him. Her boyfriend did find his much sought-after lamp there and that was that.

* * *

About a year later I was on a quest for an antique item and remembered that store. I headed back and the storeowner greeted me with an elated shout, "It's you!!" I thought he had mistaken me for someone else and he quickly regained his composure. I told him what I was looking for and he said he thought they might have something like that but he wasn't sure where. He took me on about a two-hour ramble through his store—it really was huge, but my item was not to be found. He revealed later in our courtship that he knew he didn't have it but was just stalling to keep me there as long as possible.

* * *

(* * * signify places where I actually left out some really funny details. Have to leave some material for the talk show circuit, you know.)

Fast-forward to a time in our relationship when we were sharing secrets. He revealed to me that he had "fallen in love with me at first sight" on the lamp visit and had prayed fervently every day of that whole intervening year that I would return to his store. If he hadn't blurted out "It's you!!" the day of my second visit, I might not have believed him.

So we got married and after the first two years passed during which I forbade him to broach the subject, my husband started agitating for progeny. I was in a very independent mode at the time and felt the confines of marriage were challenging enough without adding kids to the mix.

But I knew he badly wanted children and he had given me my two years. So, ambivalence notwithstanding, I went off birth control and we started trying to get pregnant.

Another two years went by and while my

husband was getting anxious, I wasn't giving it much thought. I was still totally on the fence about getting pregnant so I was willing to have it go either way.

I went to a new doc around this time. She greeted me quite briskly with, "I see from your paperwork you haven't been on any birth control for the past two years. Are you trying to get pregnant?"

I was a bit taken aback by her aggressive, confrontational attitude but responded, "Sort of. I'm a bit ambivalent on the subject."

She responded quite snidely, "Well you have nothing to worry about. You are far too fat to ever get pregnant!" Maybe it was her way of trying to inspire me to lose weight. Who knows? She wasn't the first or last doctor to try to guilt/scare me into dieting.

I was truly pretty leery about the whole pregnancy project, so far from taking her rude pronouncement badly, I found it reassuring. So reassuring in fact that I stopped worrying about the whole, Do I want to get pregnant? thing. Yep, I believed the bitch, let my psychological guards down, and two months later I was pregnant!

Fat and sassy I had a twenty-two-year marriage with all the usual ups and downs until death did us part and two magnificent, beautiful daughters who mean the world to me. I truly believe if I hadn't stopped believing FIB and learned to love myself I wouldn't have had any of that. Amen.

I'd like to close this chapter with my philosophy of life. Oddly enough, I call it my Deathbed Philosophy. Bear with me through my last mini-digression.

A friend of mine posted these words where she would see them every day:

"Nothing tastes as good as thin feels."

Words to live by? For me...not so much. If most men lead lives of quiet desperation, most women (in this culture at least) lead lives of quiet deprivation. (What the hell. Throw in desperation, too. I think there was even a TV show about that.)

My response to her saying:

Nothing feels as good as chocolate tastes. Not even sex.

I don't know about you, but chocolate has never failed to please me. Sex on the other hand...

So Death Bed Philosophy is:

Being too fat may kill you. Being too thin may kill you. Being hit by a car may kill you ad infinitum. The bottom line is we are all going to die. I decided years ago my life would never be about quantity but always about quality. (Don't get me wrong. I would happily live into my one hundreds if I could keep 90% of my marbles and a reasonable amount of independence, like say going to the bathroom without help.) This philosophy guides all my decision-making processes. Want an example? Sure you do!

I schedule a day of the week to do a much-needed chore that has needed doing for years and I am actually in the mood to do it, finally.

A friend calls and wants to get together. Nothing special, and I could easily postpone it without any hurt feelings. In fact, most of my friends would be thrilled if I took my housekeeping more seriously. So I flash-forward (hopefully wayyyyyyyy forward) to my deathbed.

Would I be thinking, "I'm so happy I cleaned my windows that day instead of having fun with my friend?"

I gotta tell you, I choose friends, fun, and food every time. I love my life!

CHAPTER 8

# *The Manifesto*

Here's what I believe:

Almost everything we are told about being fat in this country is a $FIB^2$ derived from FIB prime (Fat Is Bad).

Stressing over what others think of you and every bite of food you take definitely has an impact on your quality of life, impairing your mental and physical health. It is stress that kills, not fat.

You have to learn to love yourself to truly experience the wonder of someone else loving you. Not loving yourself is a horribly insidious state of being. It will undermine all your relationships and taint your entire life.

Based on those beliefs, here's my manifesto:

I am not a glutton.

I am not stupid.

I am not lazy.
I am not ugly.
I am not an object of scorn or ridicule. I am a person.
I am a disciplined person.
I am a smart person.
I am a person worthy of respect.
I am a person worthy of love.
I am a beautiful person inside and out.

So there you have it. My Fat Girl's Manifesto, my thin book on Living Fat in America, my Small Book on Living Large, my Ph.D. on FIB, the Ten Commandments of Cyr.

I am not trying to influence anyone else's thinking. Truly I am not, though I acknowledge that this book could. That's why I call it *A Fat Girl's Manifesto,* not "The Fat Girl's Manifesto." It really is all about me...my experiences and the conclusions to which they overwhelmingly have led me.

Having now read this book, you might decide it is utter nonsense. If, on the other hand, these pages got a big fat "YES!!" (smile when you read the words "big fat,"—I am) out of you deep in your being, I hope you can release any stress and negativity you have about being fat and live a fierce, fearless, and fabulous life.

It probably wouldn't hurt to move to Tahiti either. I'd love to meet you there!

# *Bibliography*

Angell, Marcia. Kassirer, Jerome P. 1998. "Losing Weight: An Ill-fated New Year's Resolution." *The New England Journal of Medicine*. 338:52-54

Emerson, Ralph Waldo. URL: www.goodreads.com/quotes/876-to-be-yourself-in-a-world-that-is-constantly-trying

Fitzgerald, Faith. 1981. "The Problem of Obesity." *Annual Review of Medicine*. 32:221-231

Gaesser, Glenn A. 2002. *Big Fat Lies: The Truth About Your Weight and Your Health*. Carlsbad (CA): Gurze Books

Gardner, Amanda. 2012. "Many Obese Americans Struggle with Stigma, Discrimination, Polls Find." *Health Day*. URL: http://consumer.healthday.com/vitamins-and-nutritional-information-27/obesity-health-news-505/many-obese-americans-struggle-with-stigma-discrimination-poll-finds-667697.html

Johnson, Jone Lewis."Eleanor Roosevelt Quotes."About Women's History. URL: http://womenshistory.about.com/cs/quotes/qu_e_roosevelt.htm

Mann, George V. 1971. "Obesity, the Nutritional Spook." *American Journal of Public Health*. 61:1491-1498

Miles, Kathleen. 2013. "Fat Genes" Determine Obesity, UCLA Study Says, In Addition to Diet and Exercise." *The Huffington Post*. URL: www.huffingtonpost.com/2013/01/10/fat-genes-obesity-ucla-study-diet-exercise_n_2450108.html

National Center for Injury Prevention and Control. CDC Injury Research Agenda. Atlanta (GA): Centers for Disease Control and Prevention; 2002

Rosen, Peg. 2013. "Can You be Fit but Fat?" *Fitness Magazine*. URL: www.fitnessmagazine.com/health/body/head-to-toe/fat-but-fit/

Sifferlin, Alexandria. 2013. "New Genes ID'd in Obesity: How Much of Weight is Genetic?" *Time*. URL: www.healthland.time.com/2013/07/19/news-genes-idd-in-obesity-how-much-of-weight-is-genetic/

Winterburn, Steven. URL: https://twitter.com/5tevenw/status/73091190475595776

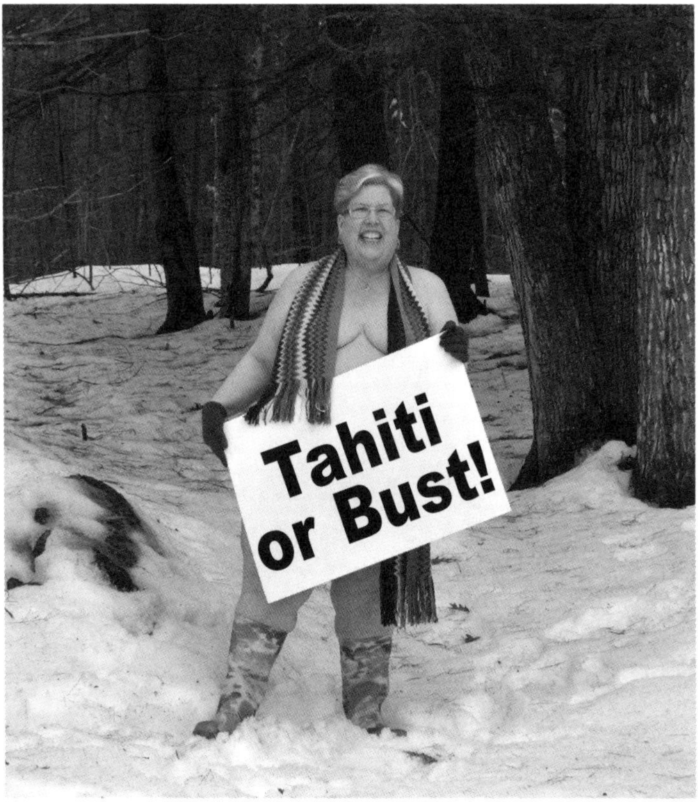
Tahiti
or Bust!

# *About the Author*

As if I haven't told you (and shown you) more than enough already, right? But in keeping with my philosophy of More is More, here's... well... more!

I was born and raised in Dayton, Ohio. While attending Bennington College I fell in love with the Northeast first and my husband second. I moved to New Hampshire with my husband's job and for thirty years have lived and worked in the town of New Boston where I've raised my two amazing daughters.

I have led many lives in my sixty-three years on this planet: Teacher, Artist, Postal Worker, Proofreader, Activist, and most importantly Mother to the aforementioned fantastic daughters. With my sixties upon me and my girls grown I decided to try out the Writing Life. The resulting book, A Fat Girl's Manifesto (A thin book on living FAT in America), addresses an issue that plagued my entire life, living in a country having a war on obesity.

# *The "Skinny" on the About the Author Photo*

OK. Here's what you absolutely *must* know about that picture. It is the result of an amazingly brilliant and completely hilarious collaboration between four utterly fabulous women:

Deb Muir – Photographer
Jen Brown – Graphic Artist
Kim Cahill – Hair and Make-up Artist
and of course
Me!!

You need to know it was taken in Kim's backyard on March 29, 2014! Yup, still well over a foot of snow on the ground more than a week into spring, but a pleasant 47 degrees out so being naked in the snow wasn't too bad. Falling down naked in the snow was another story altogether and proved far too racy to document on film.

Thank you Deb, Jen, and Kim for one of the most terrifically fun experiences of my life! And a special thanks to Marty (Kim's husband) for being such a good sport about letting a crazy naked lady hijack his wife and his home for five hours or so on what otherwise would have been a quiet, peaceful Saturday.